Patterns for Mindfulness
Volume 1

31 Square & Rectangle Patterns to Color

Adult Coloring Book for Relief from Stress, Anxiety & Depression

By Nerine Martin
ColorYourWayToHappy.com

Cover and Book Design by Nerine Martin

Copyright 2019 Nerine Martin. All rights reserved.

www.ColorYourWayToHappy.com

Preview of Designs

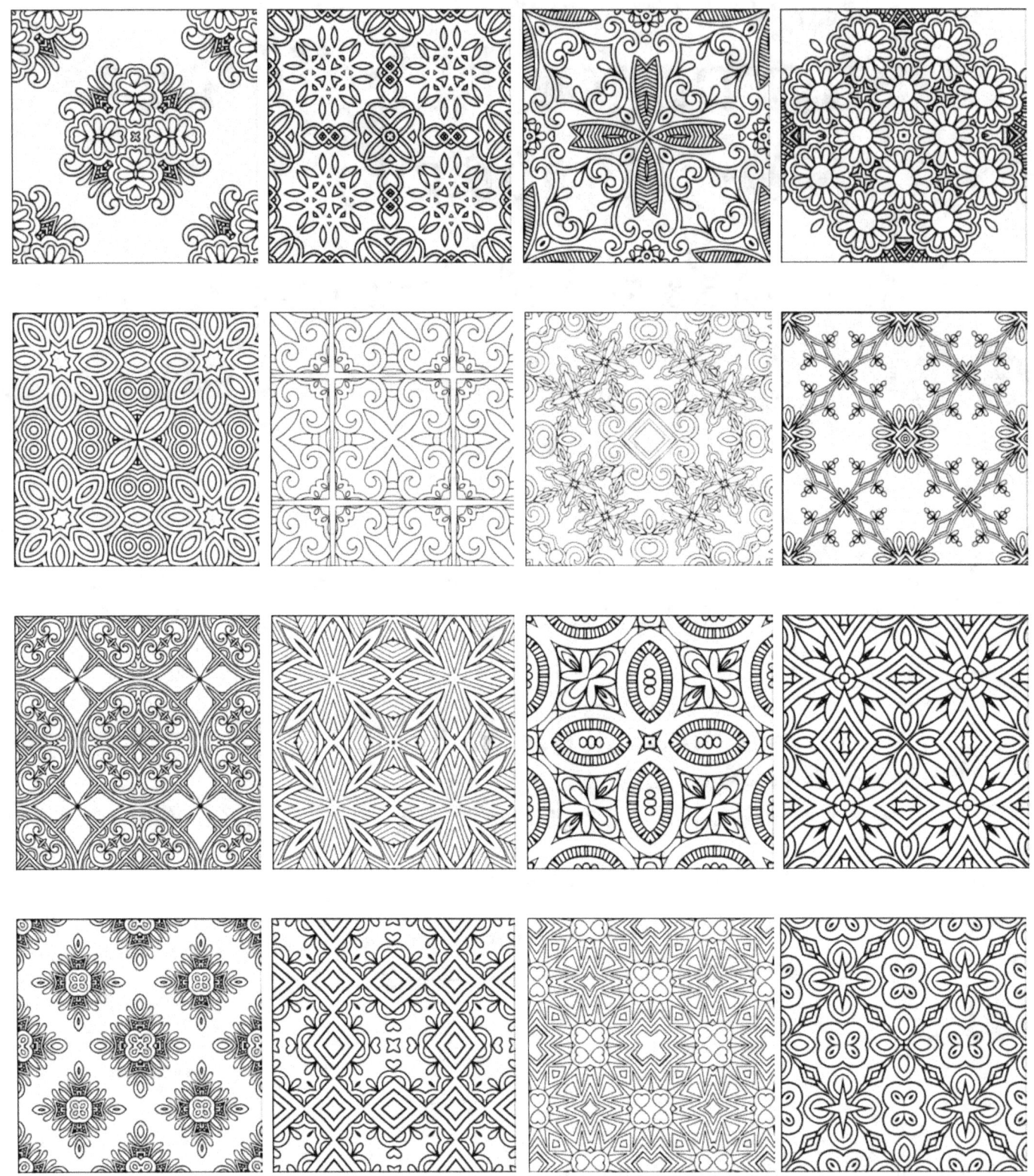

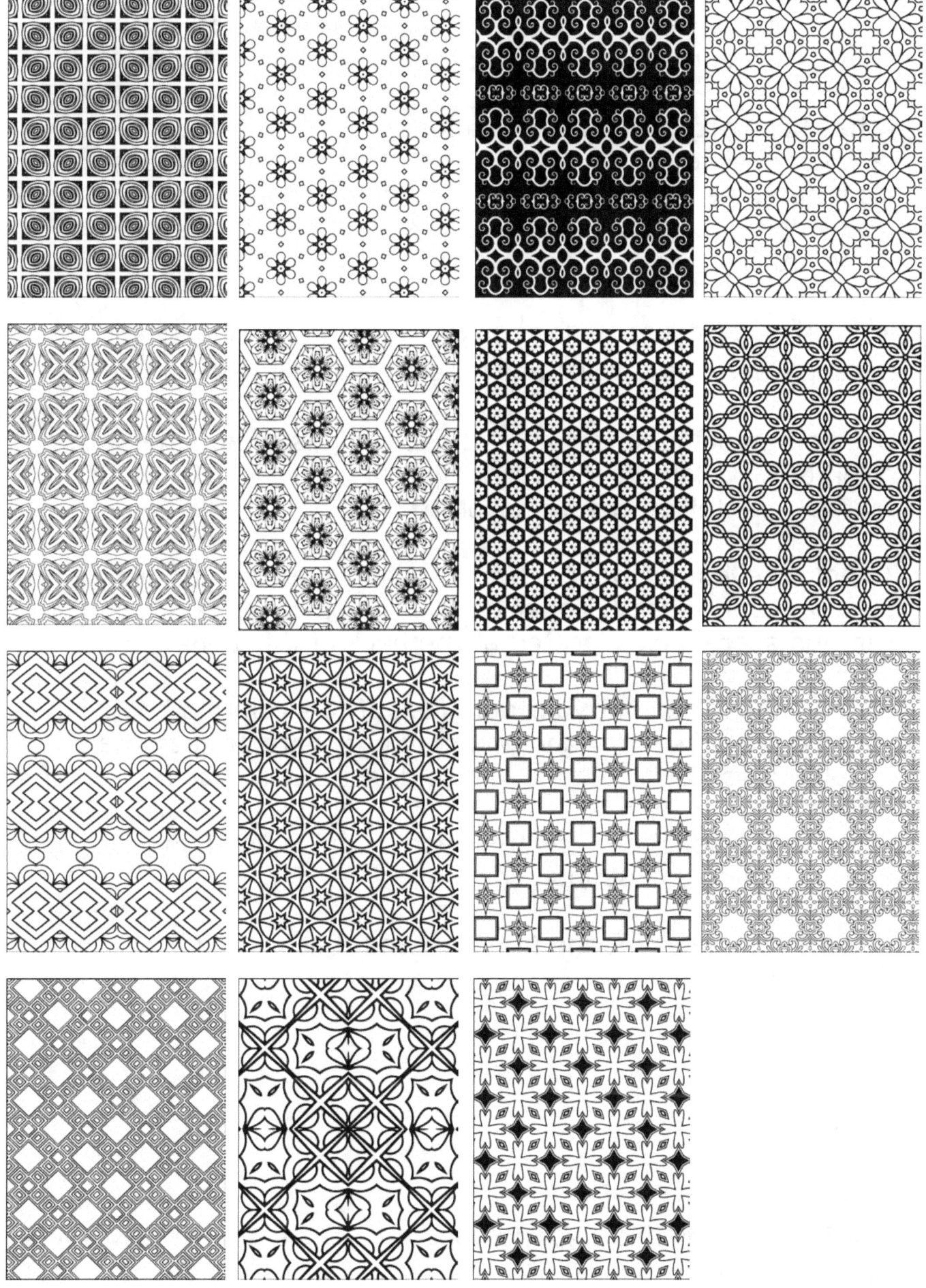

Congratulations on your purchase of *Patterns for Mindfulness Volume 1* and thank you for choosing my coloring book.

It has been proven that using coloring as a form of art therapy, can help relieve symptoms of stress, anxiety and depression by distracting the mind's thought processes. Coloring can also aid as a coping strategy to get through those difficult times, such as a panic attack.

Inside this gorgeous coloring book, you will find 31 square and rectangle patterns to color, one for every day of the month!

Use your imagination to make these designs come alive with color, using colored pencils, felt tip markers, gel pens, fluoro markers, metallic pens or crayons.

To help prevent any bleed through when using felt tip markers – place a blank sheet of paper behind the page when coloring. You can find spare pages located at the back of this book.

Please remember that your purchase of this coloring book is for your personal use only and you may not share or copy the uncolored pages for others. Please direct other people to purchase their own copy. By doing so, you are supporting my art so I can continue to make more coloring books and I thank you for your understanding and support. ☺

I hope you enjoy coloring my book and that you 'Color Your Way To Happy'.

Yours in coloring,

Nerine ☺

P.S. If you enjoy this coloring book, please be so kind to leave a review on Amazon.

Use This Area To Test Your Colors

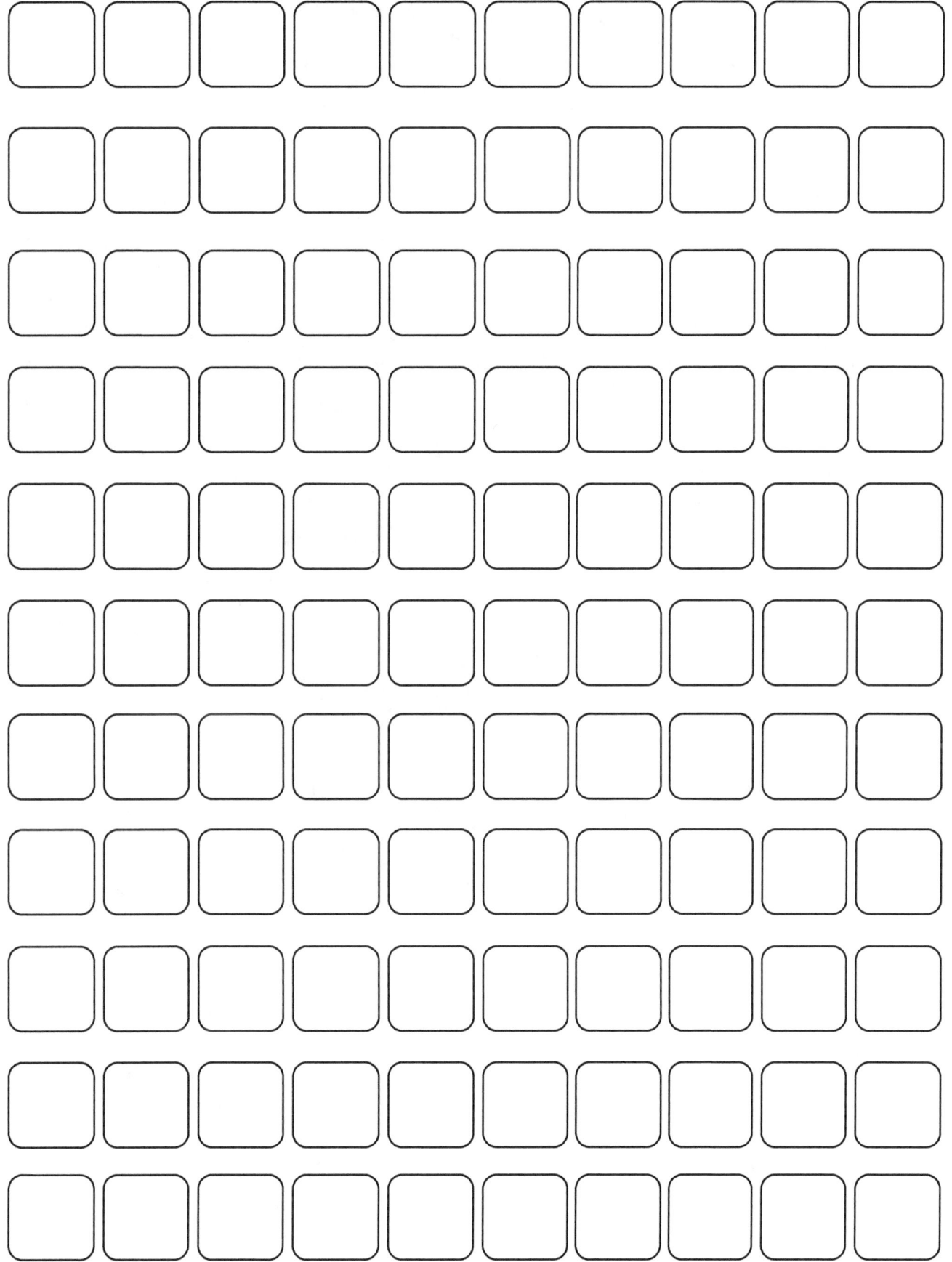

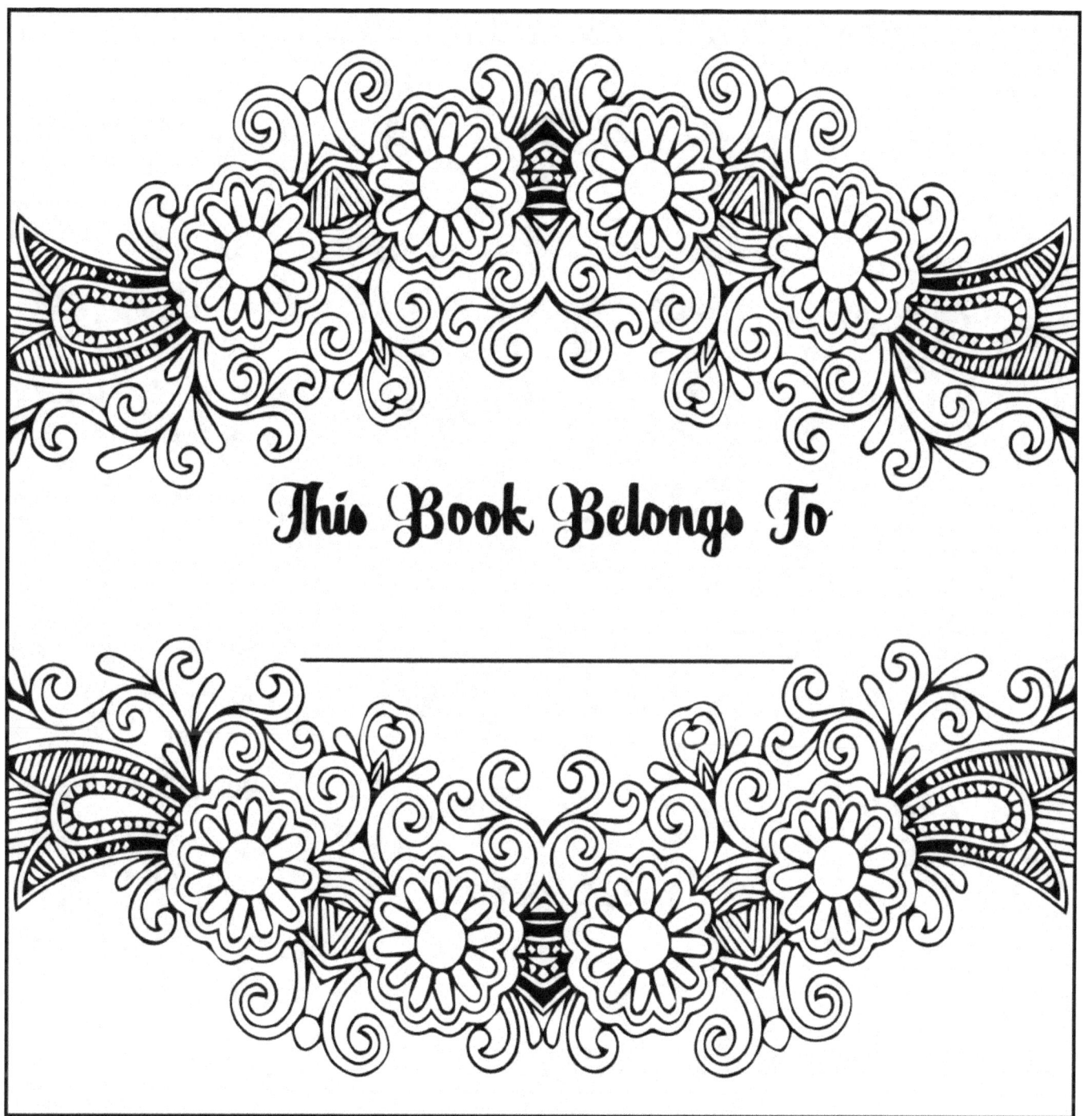

This Book Belongs To

_____

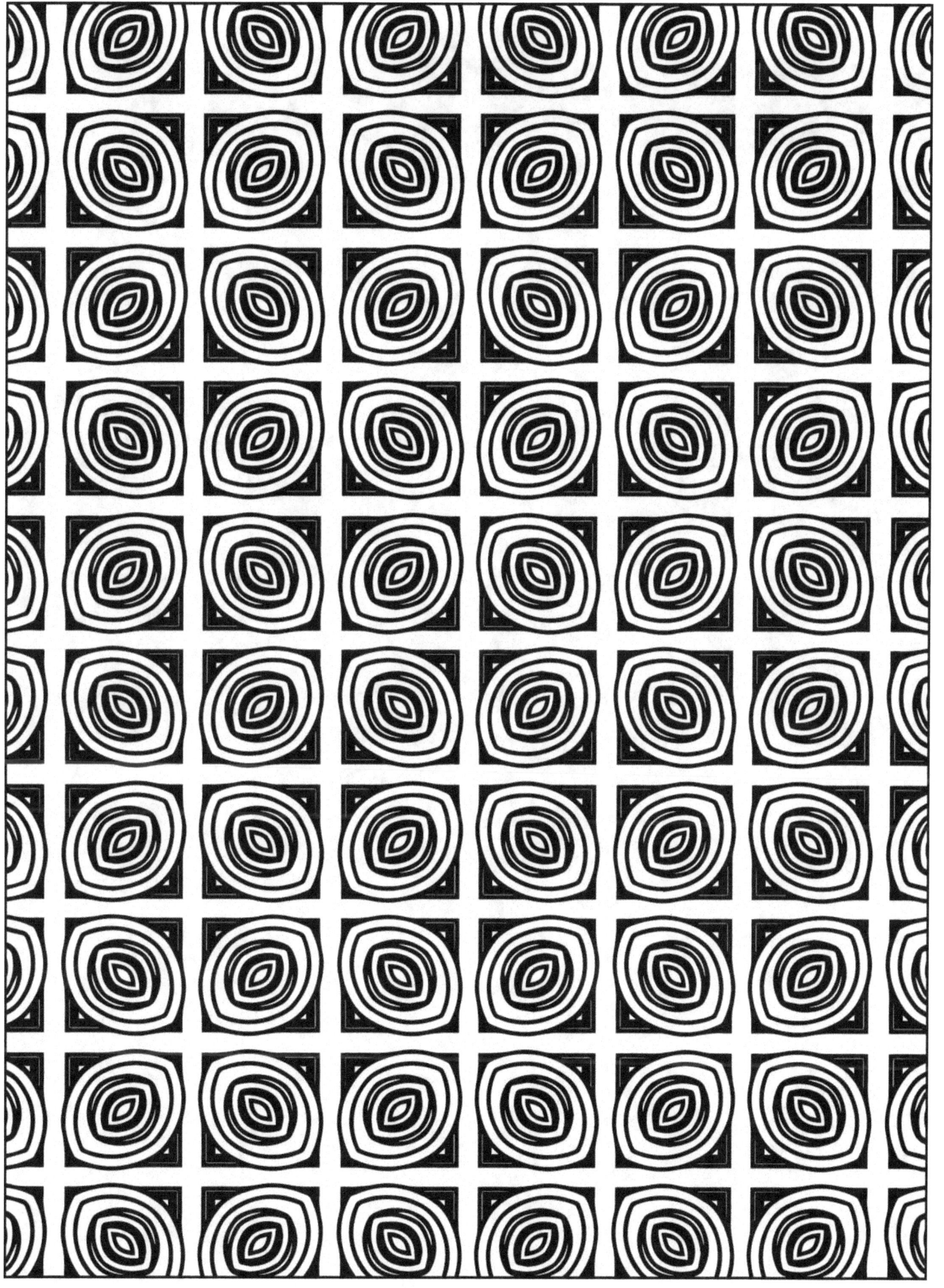

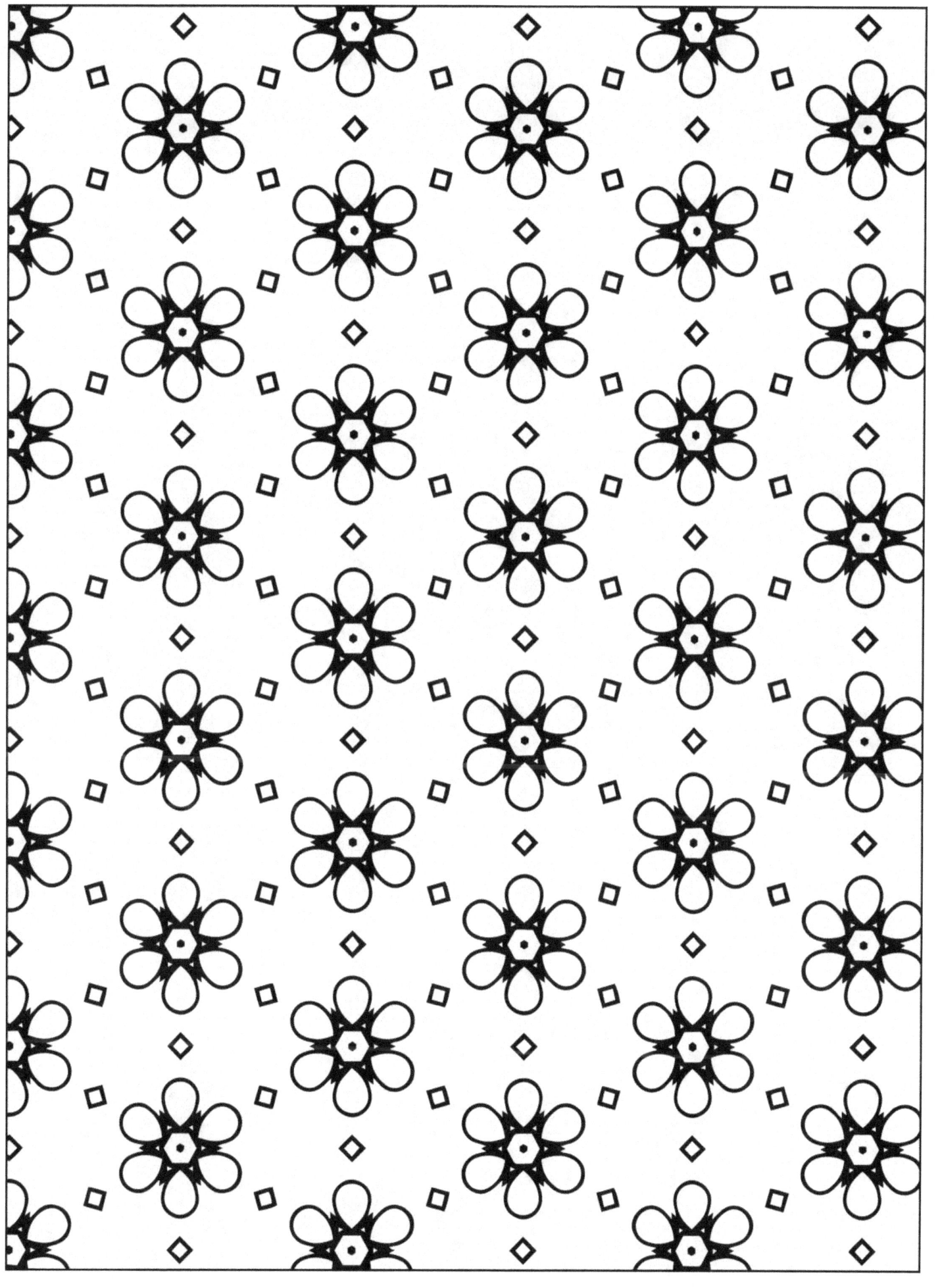

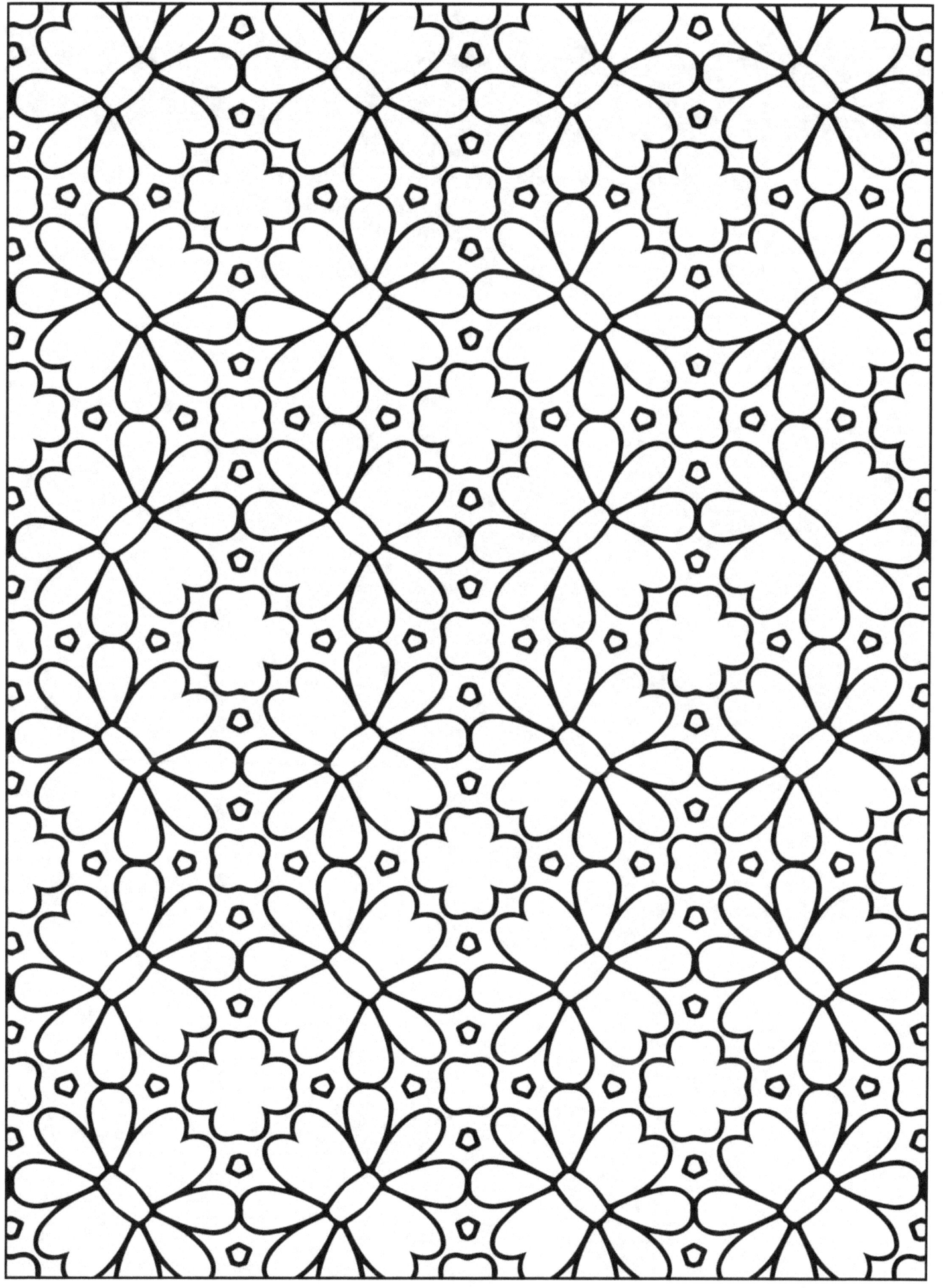

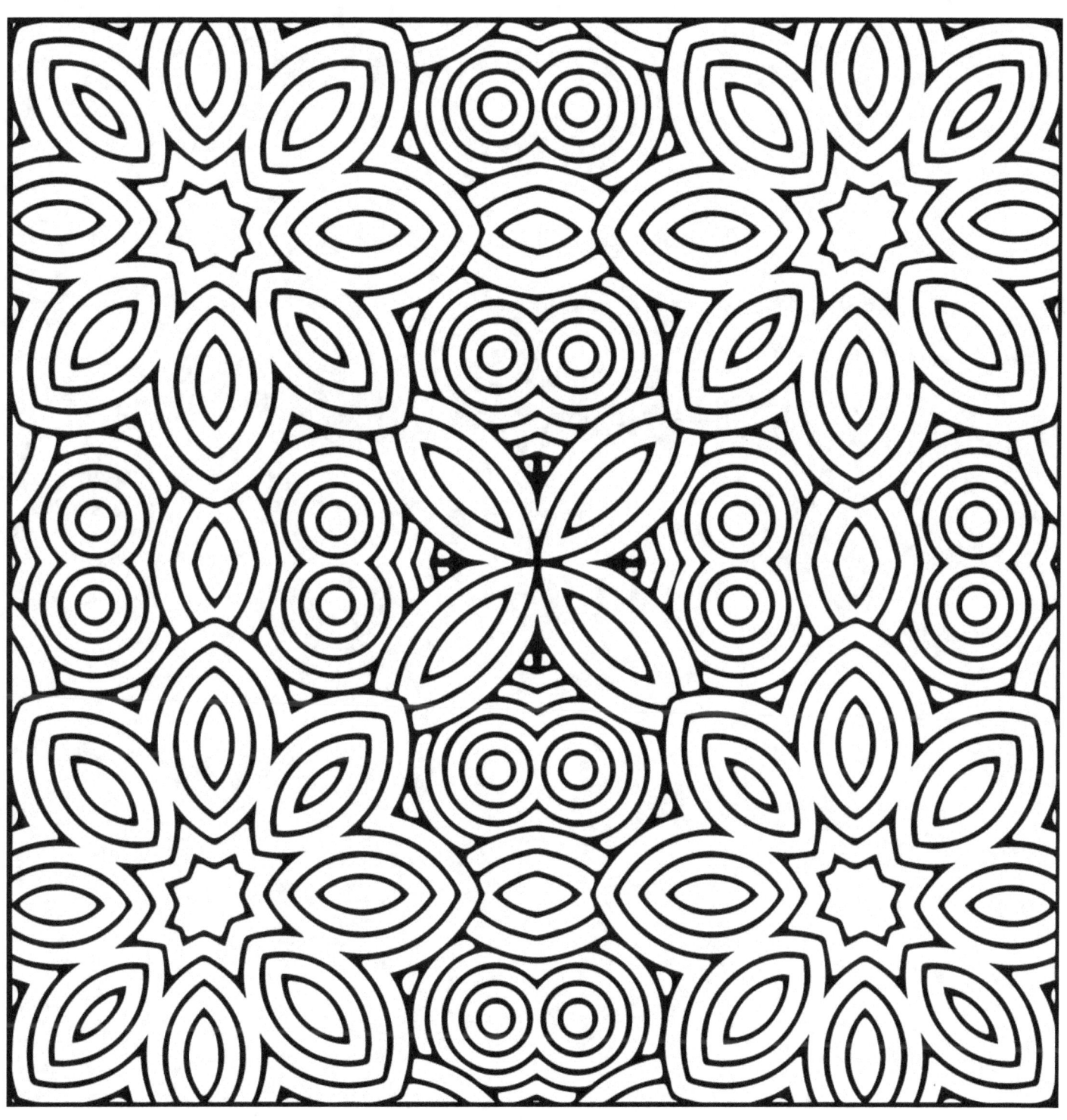

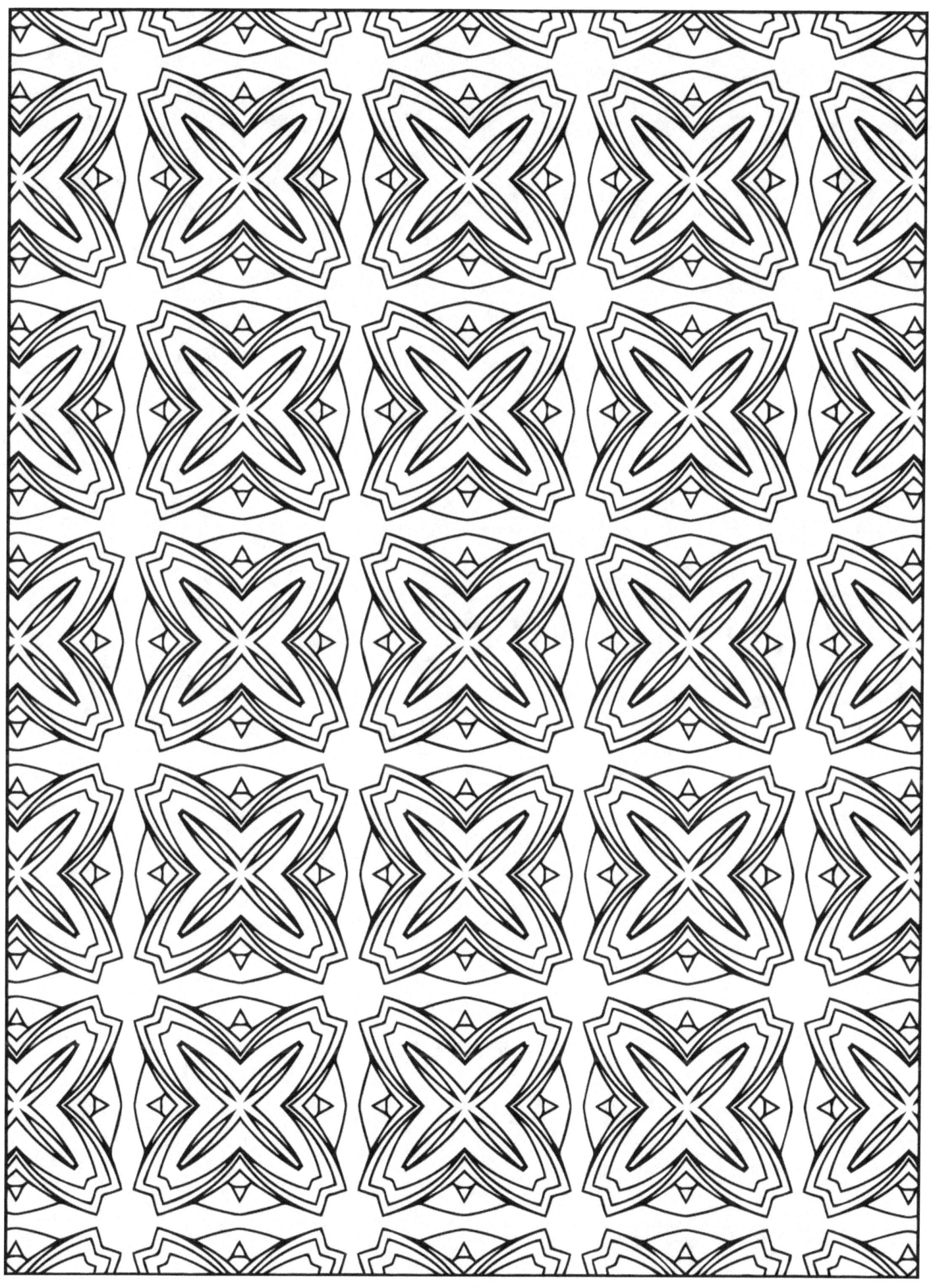

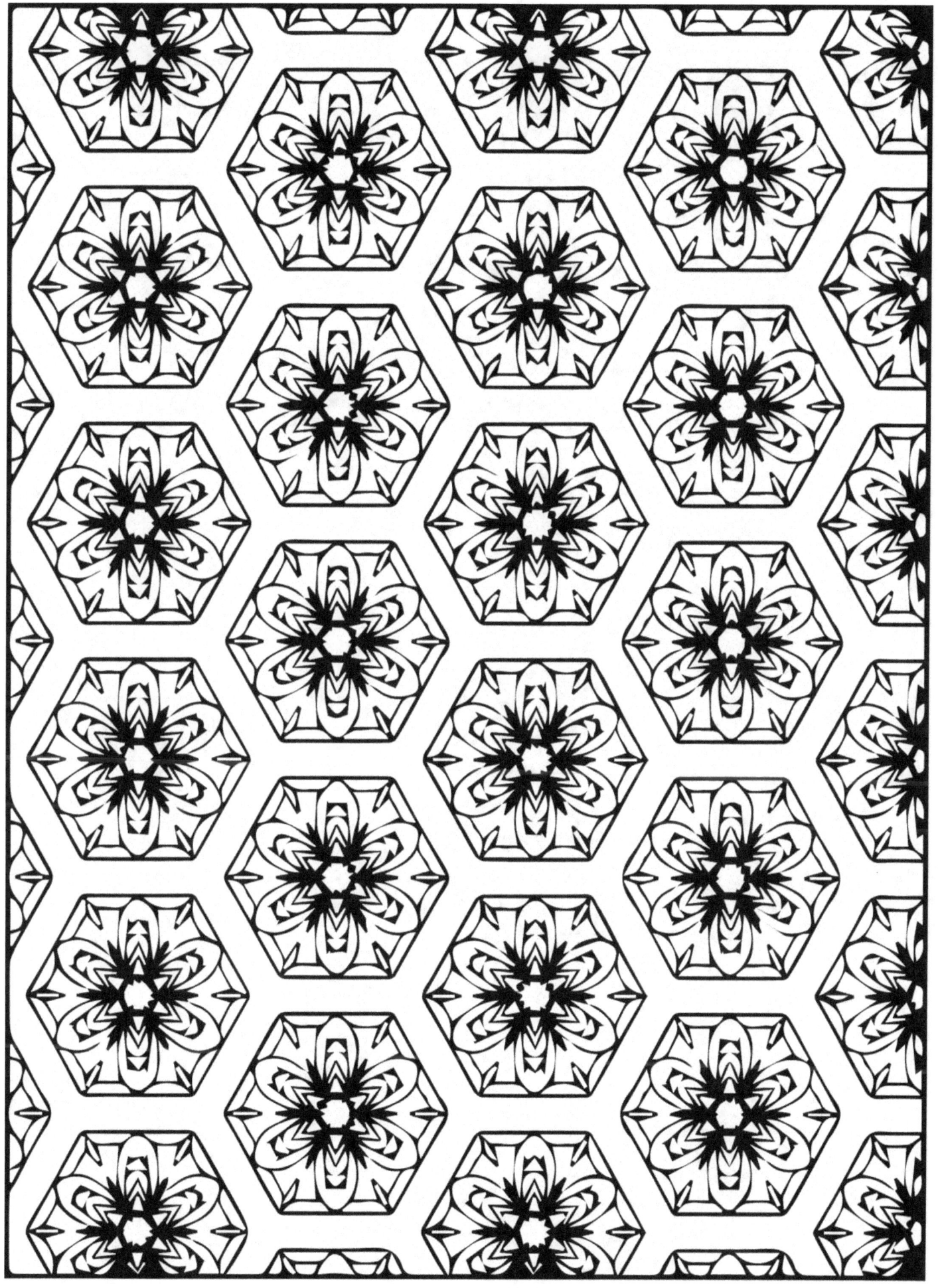

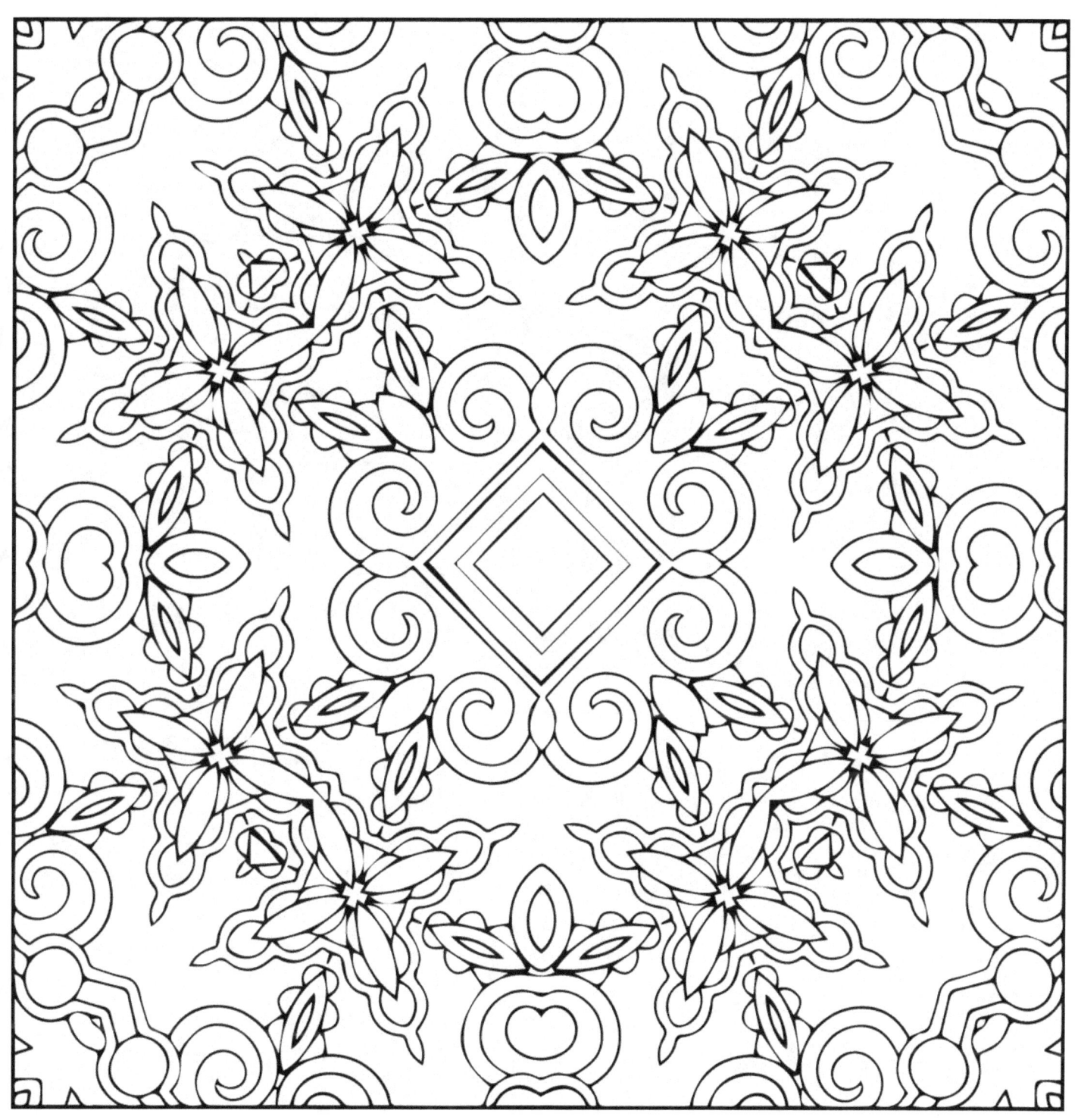

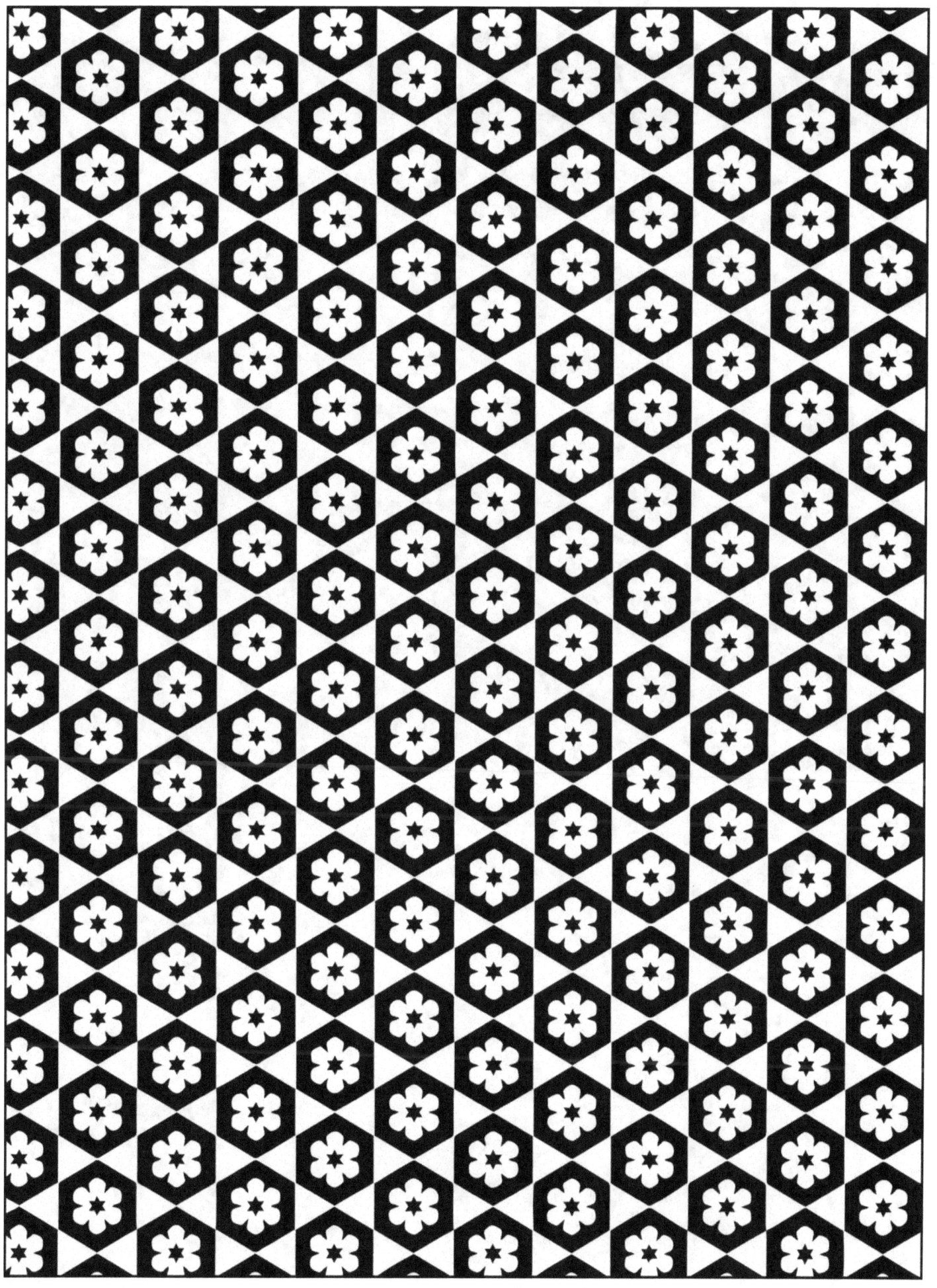

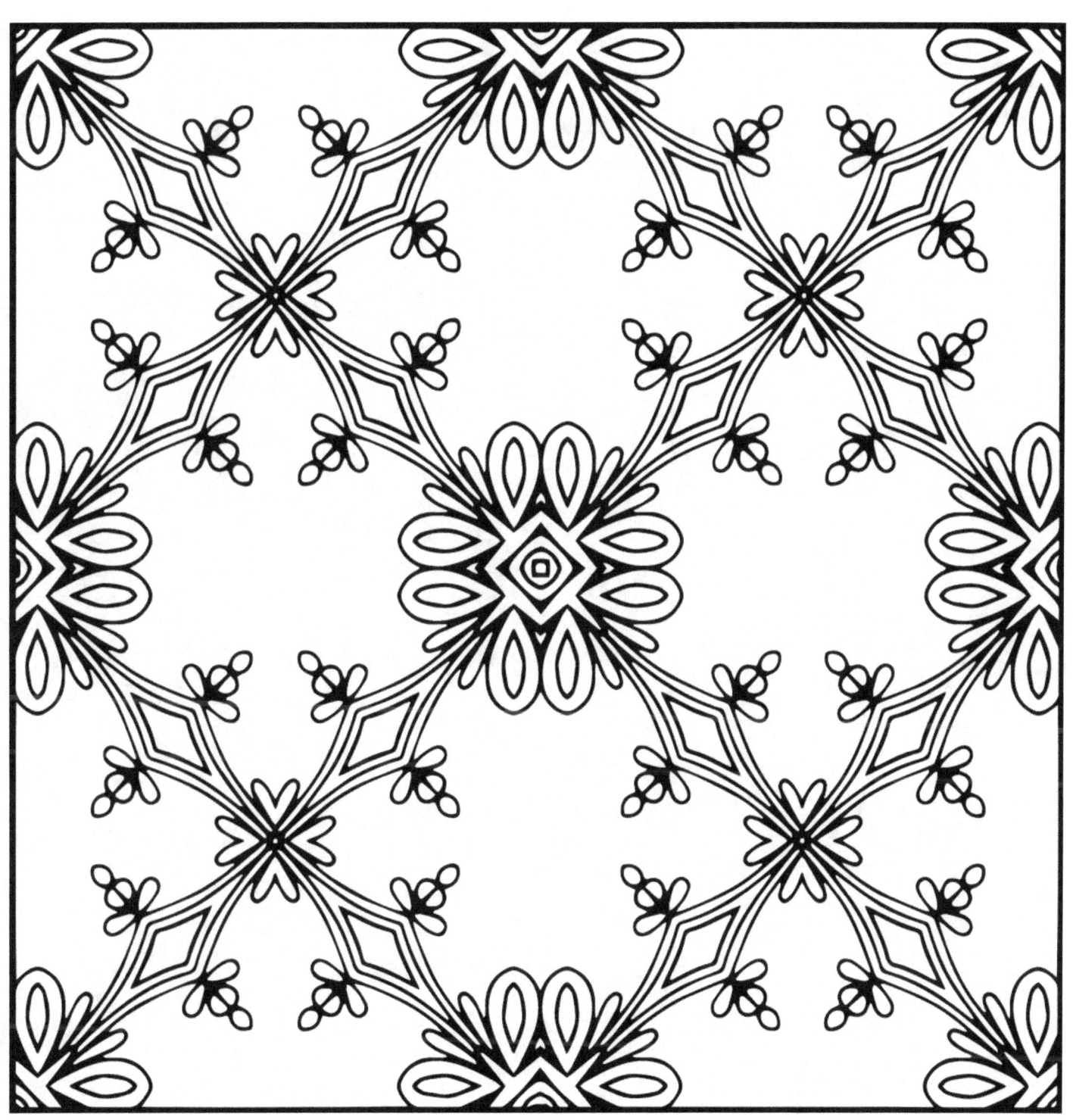

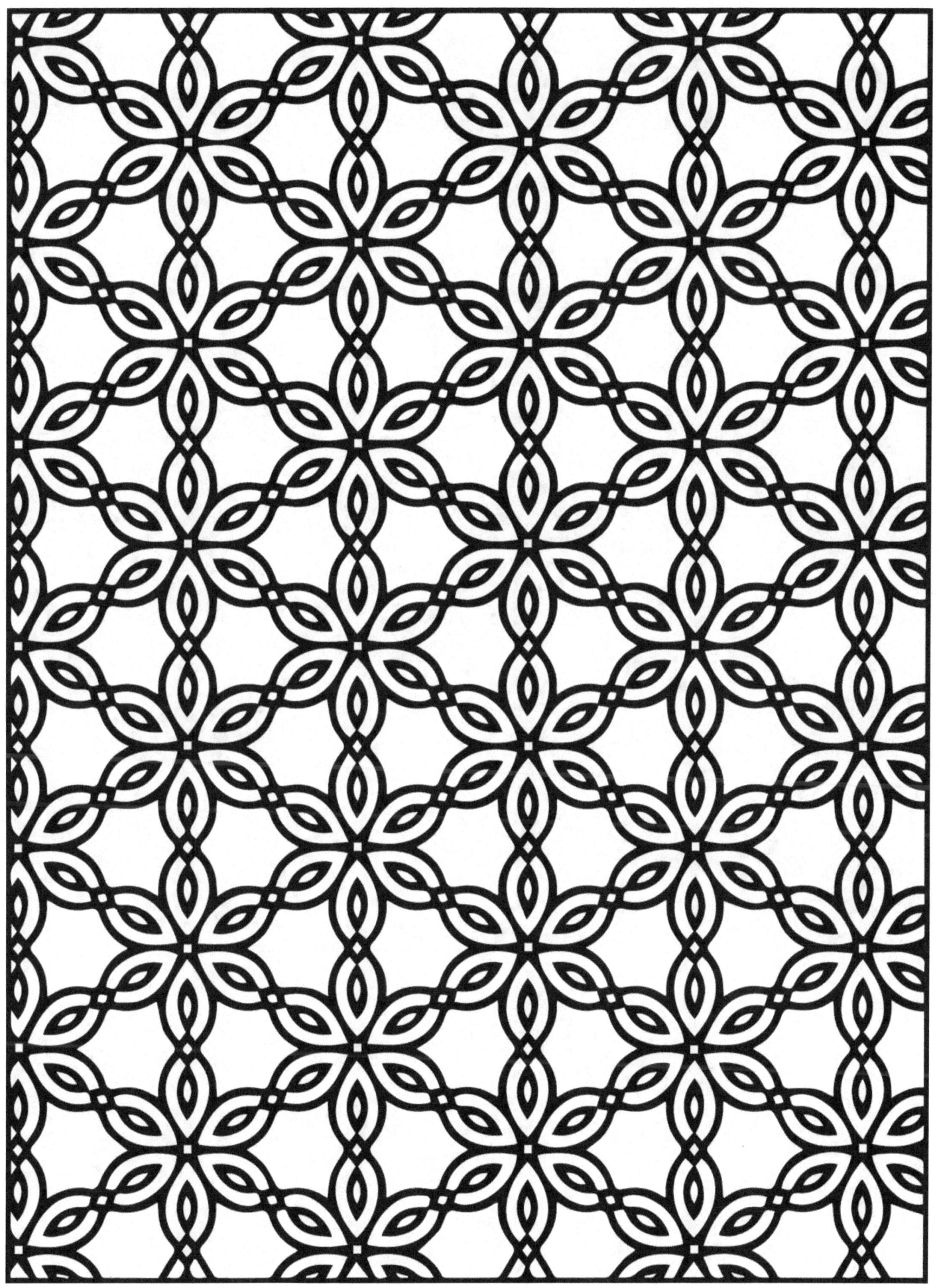

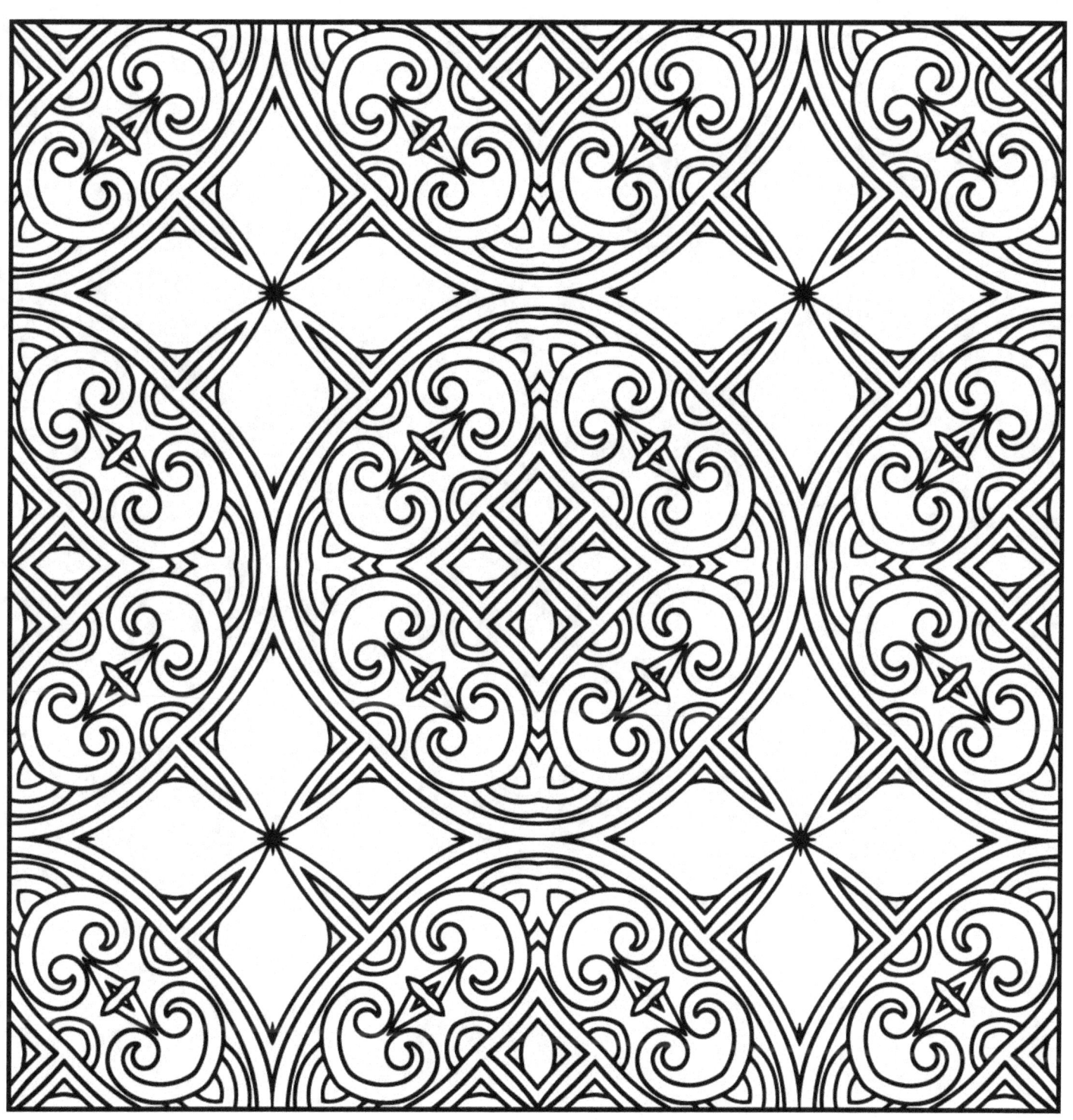

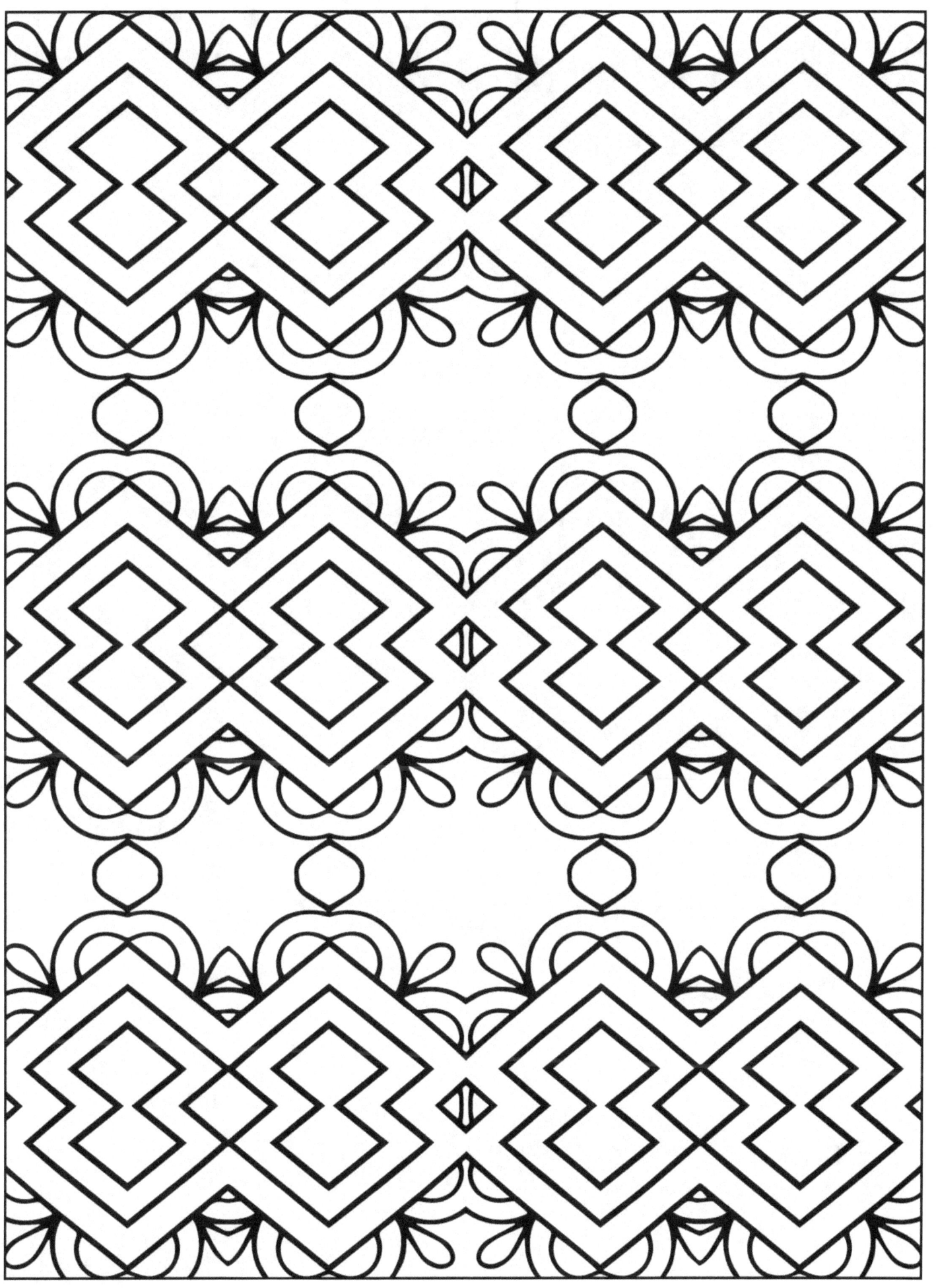

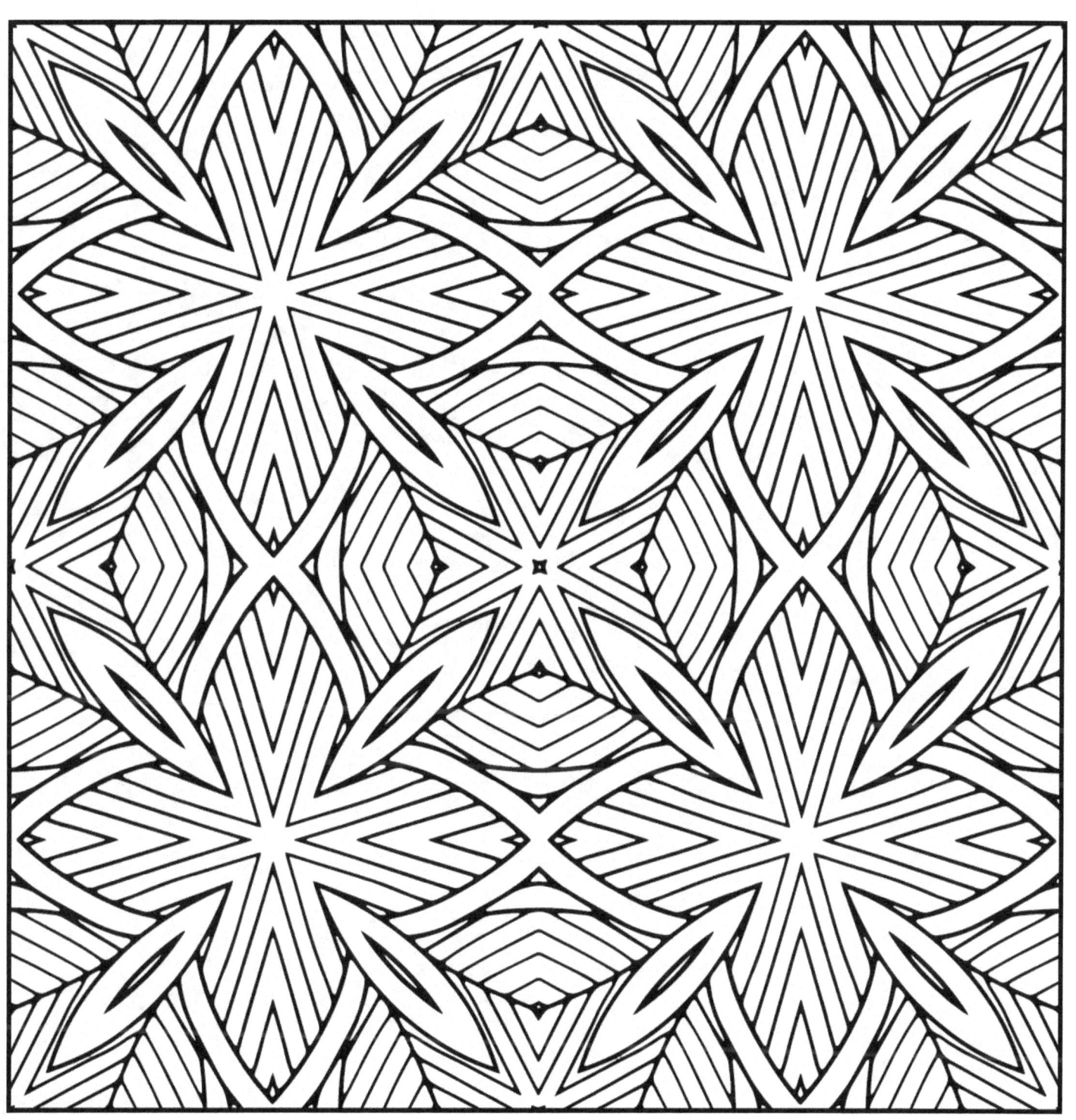

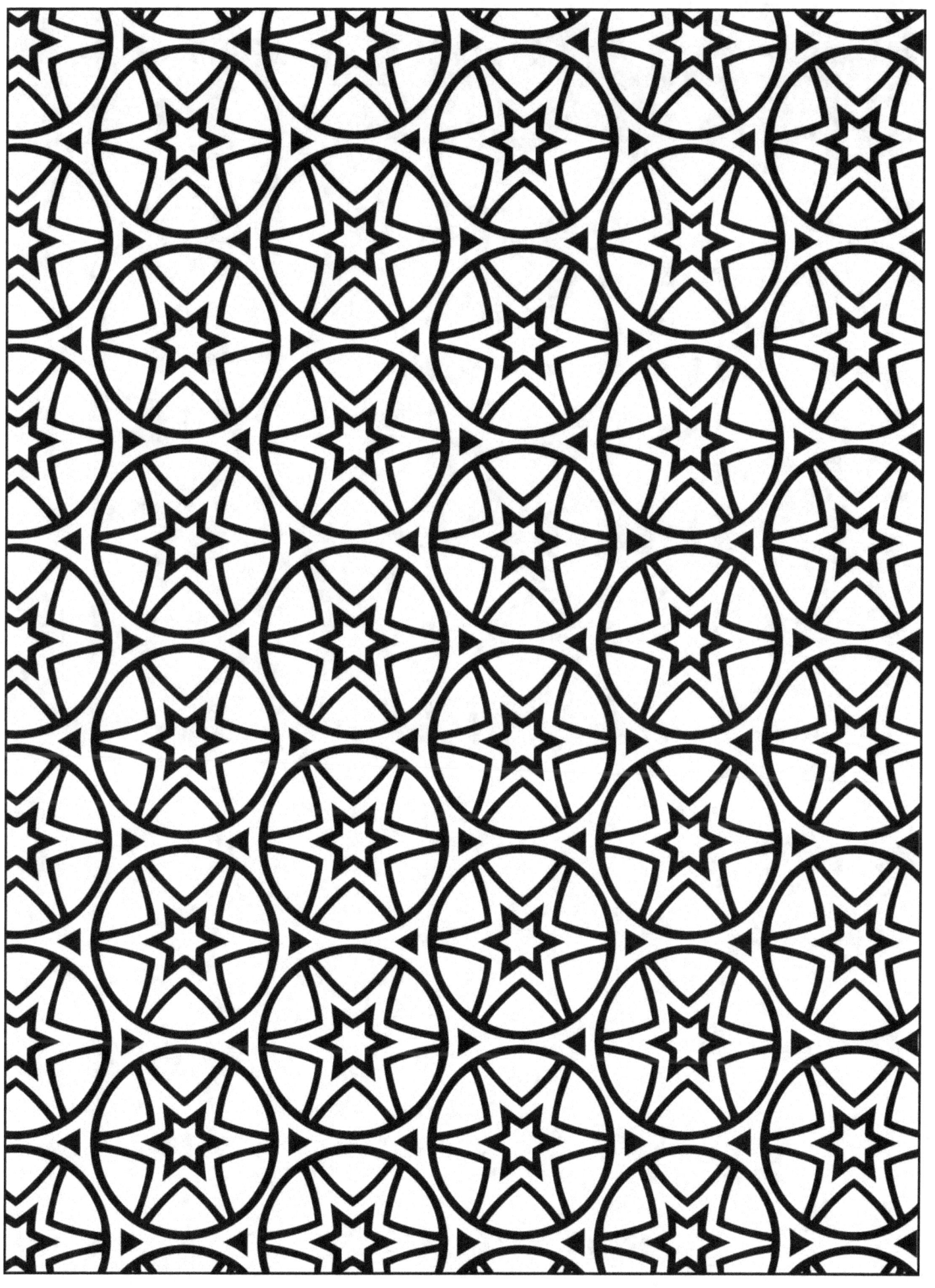

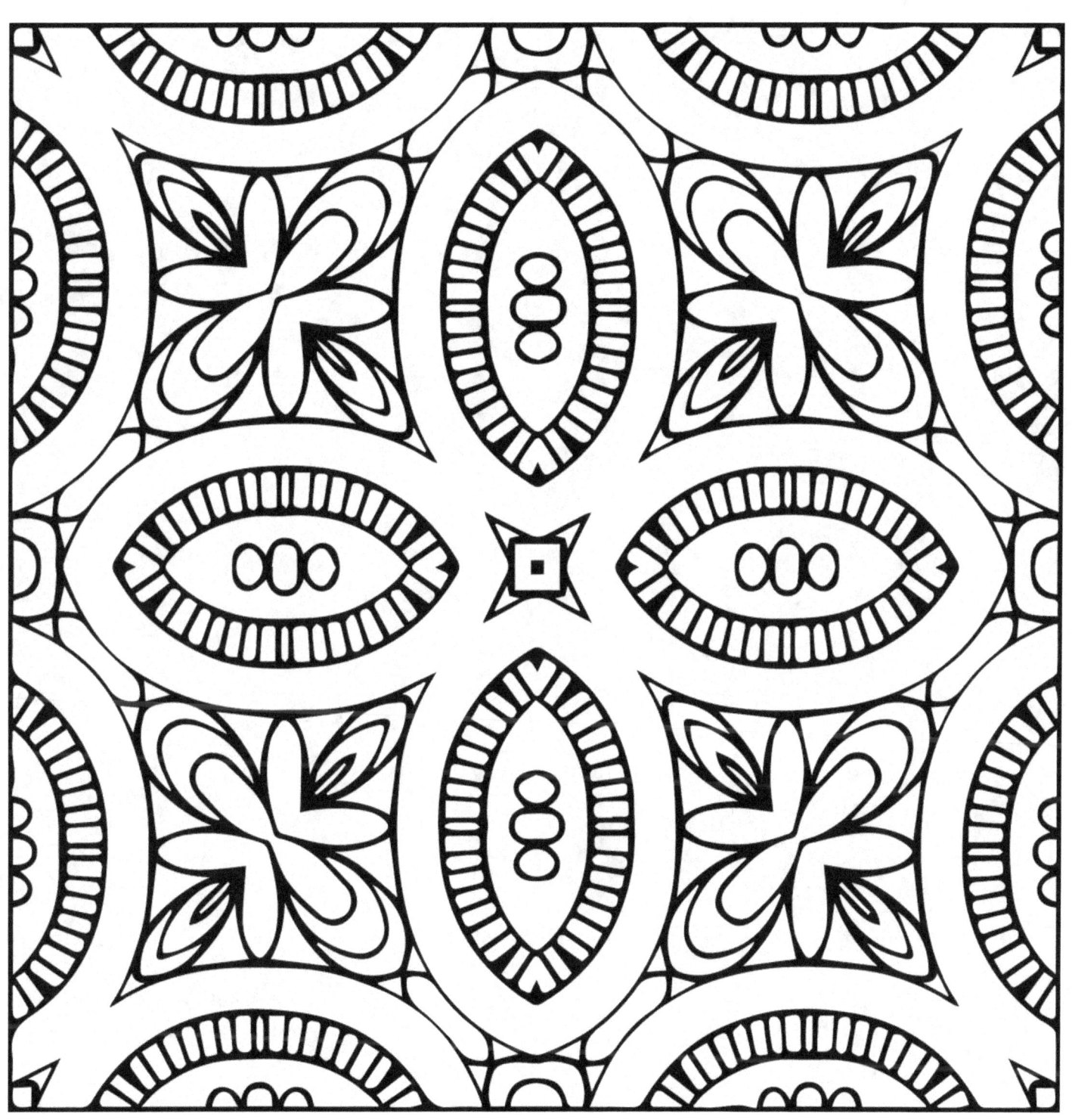

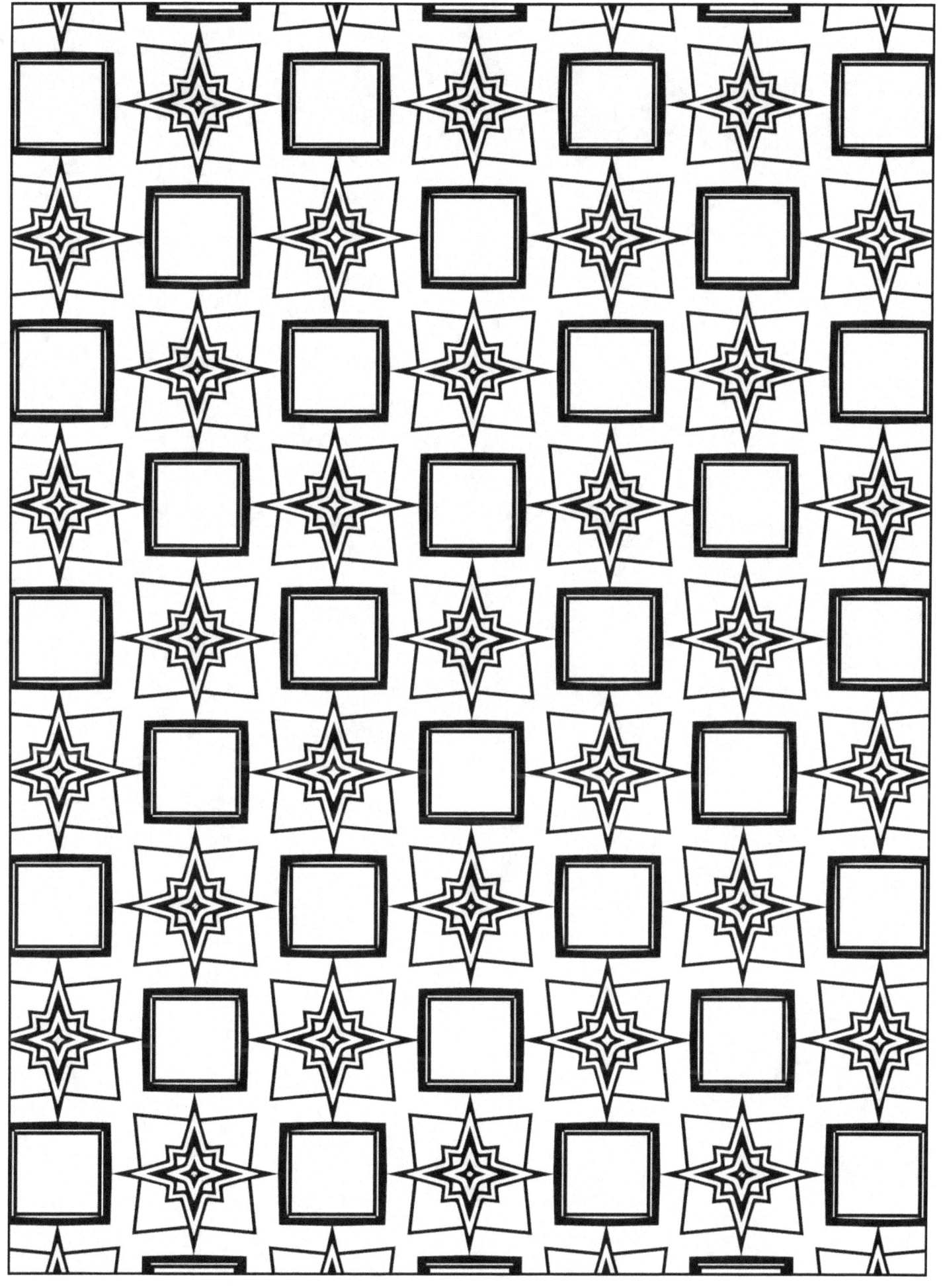

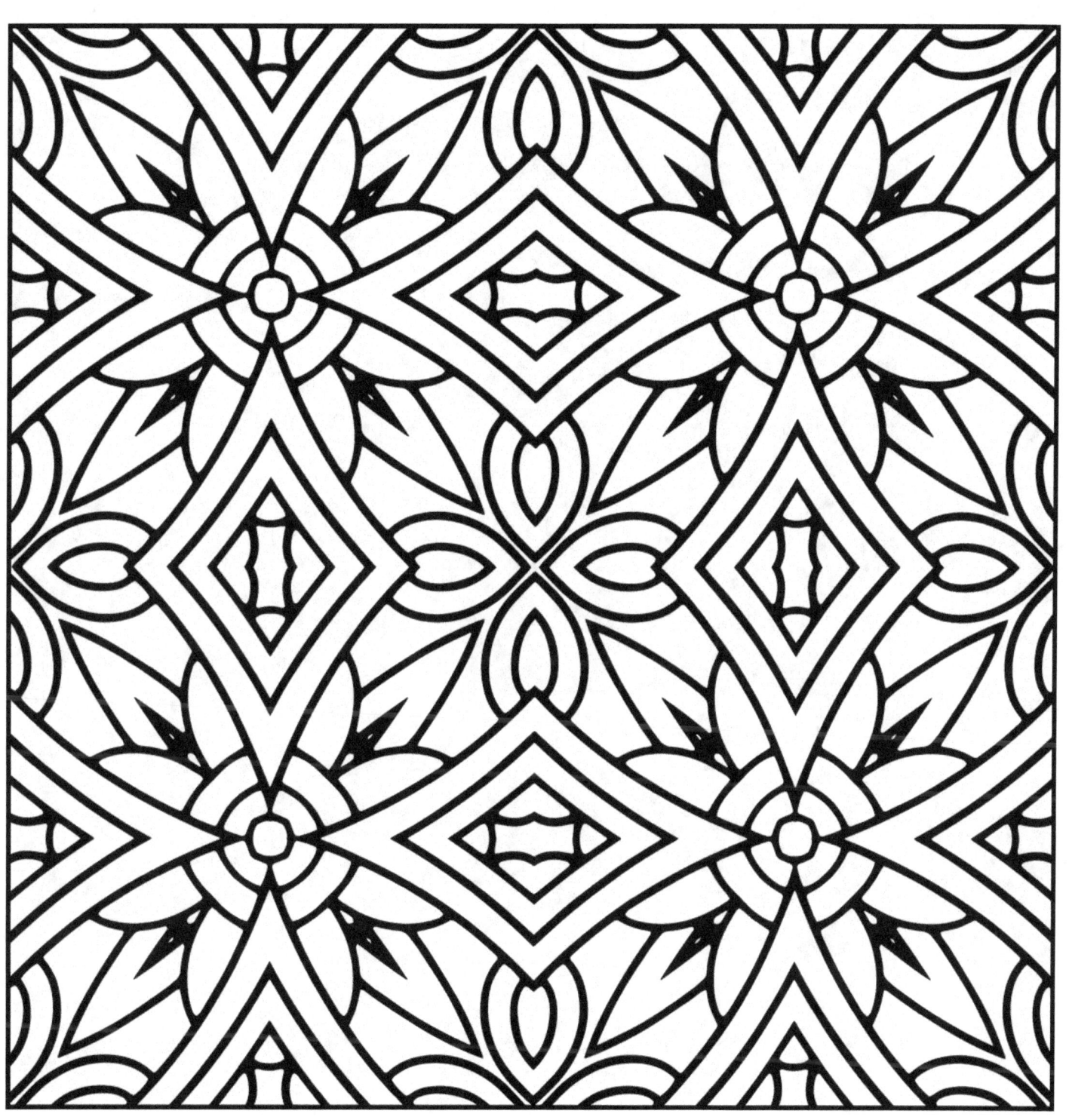

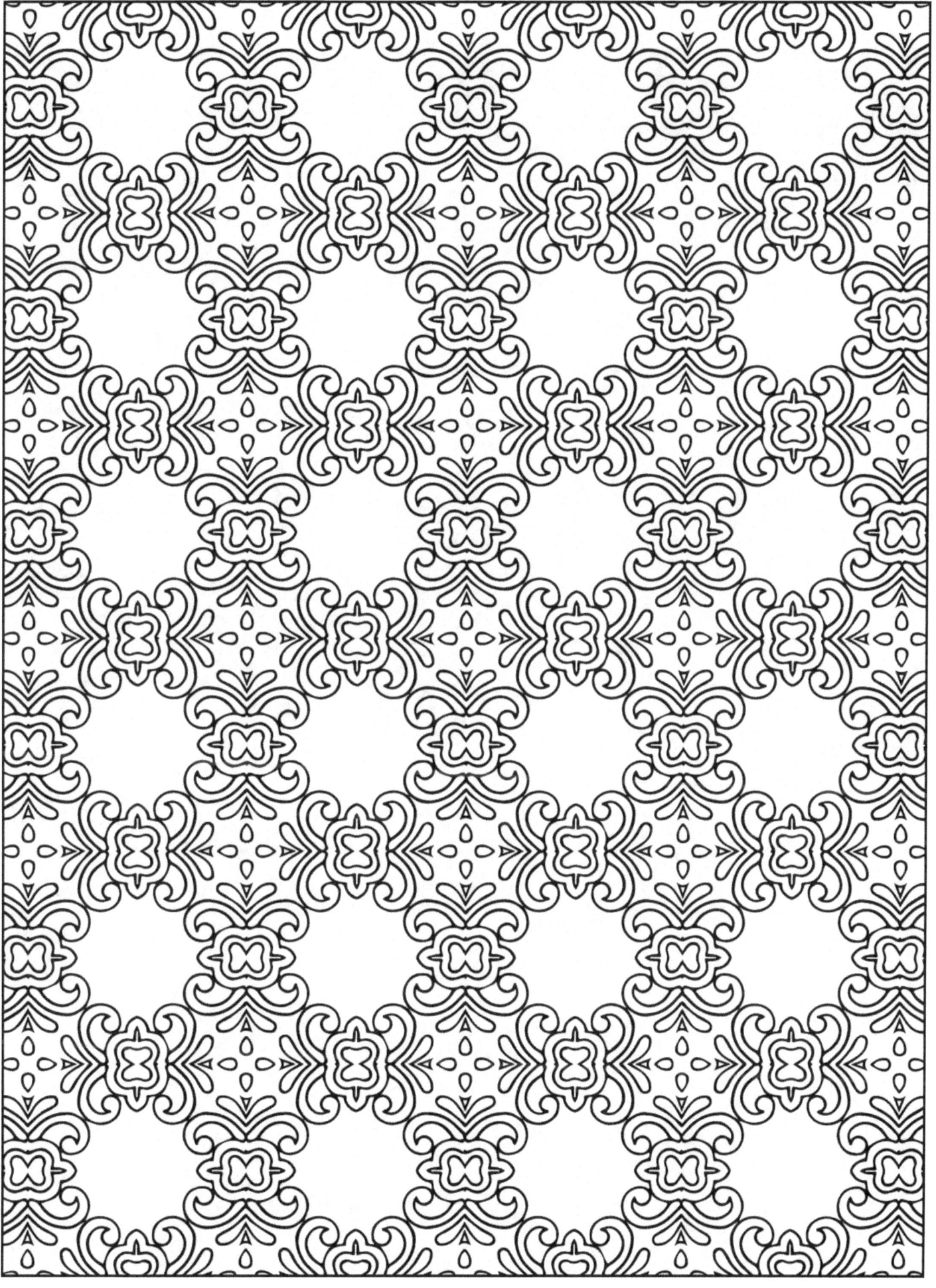

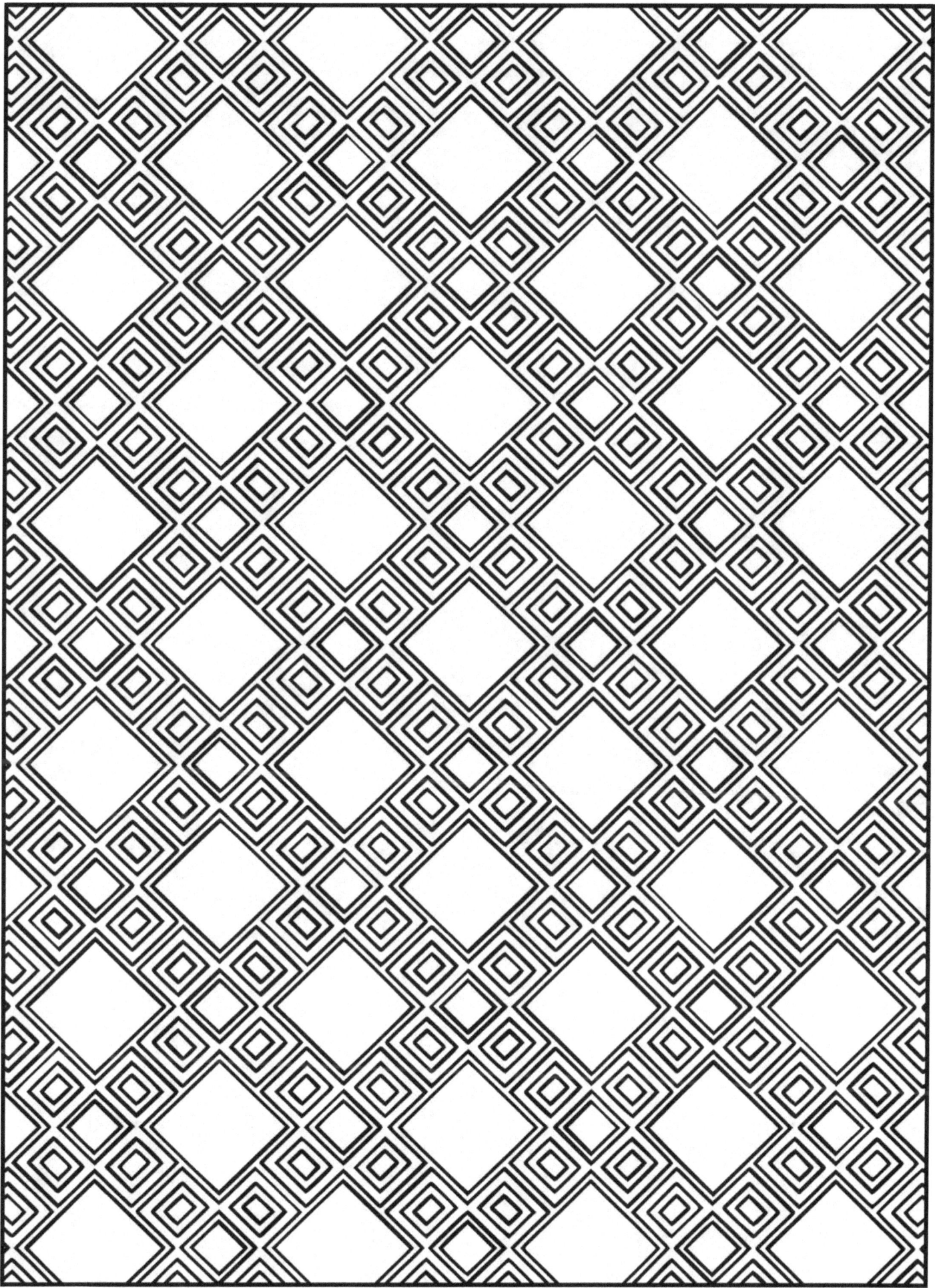

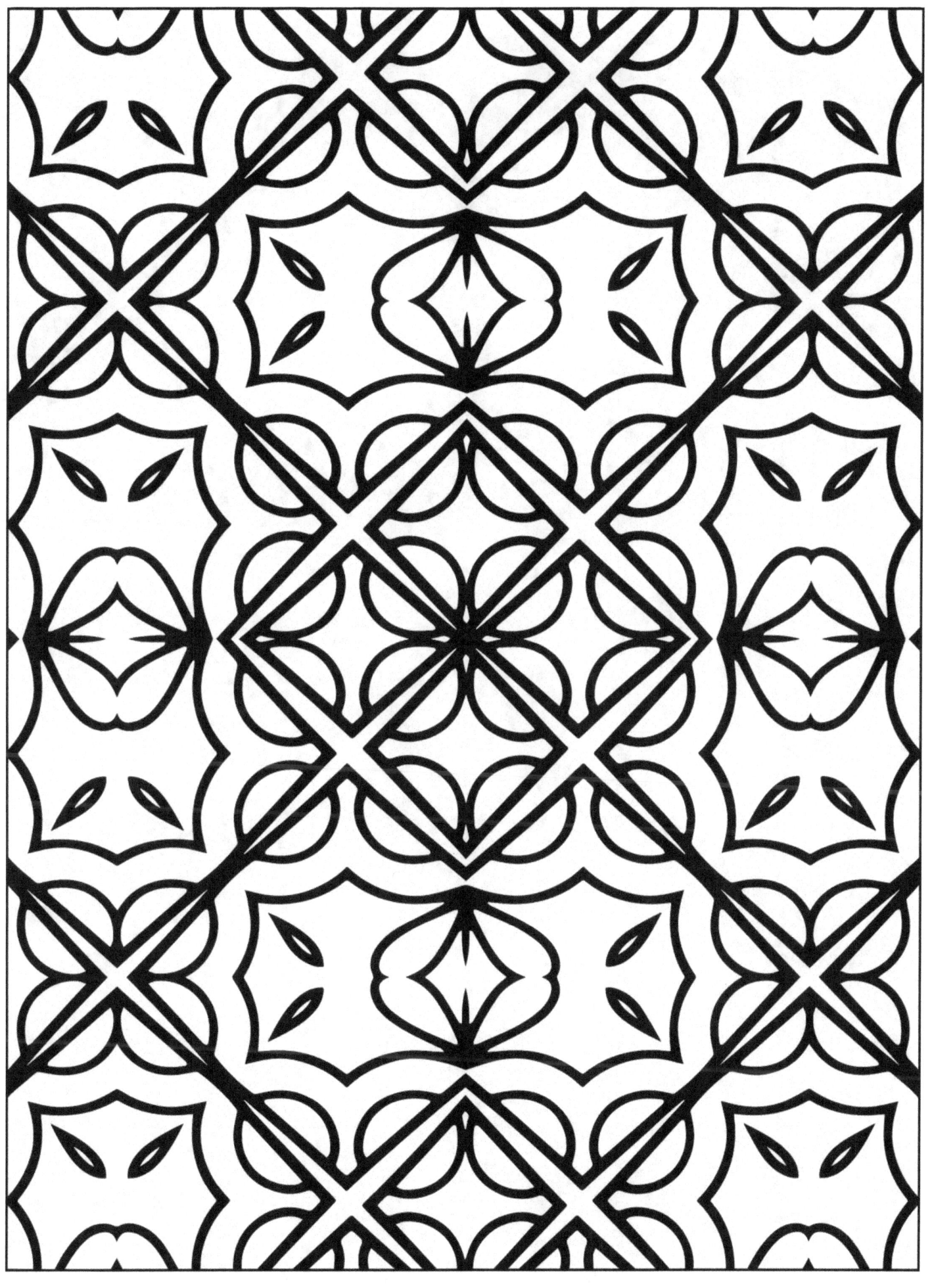

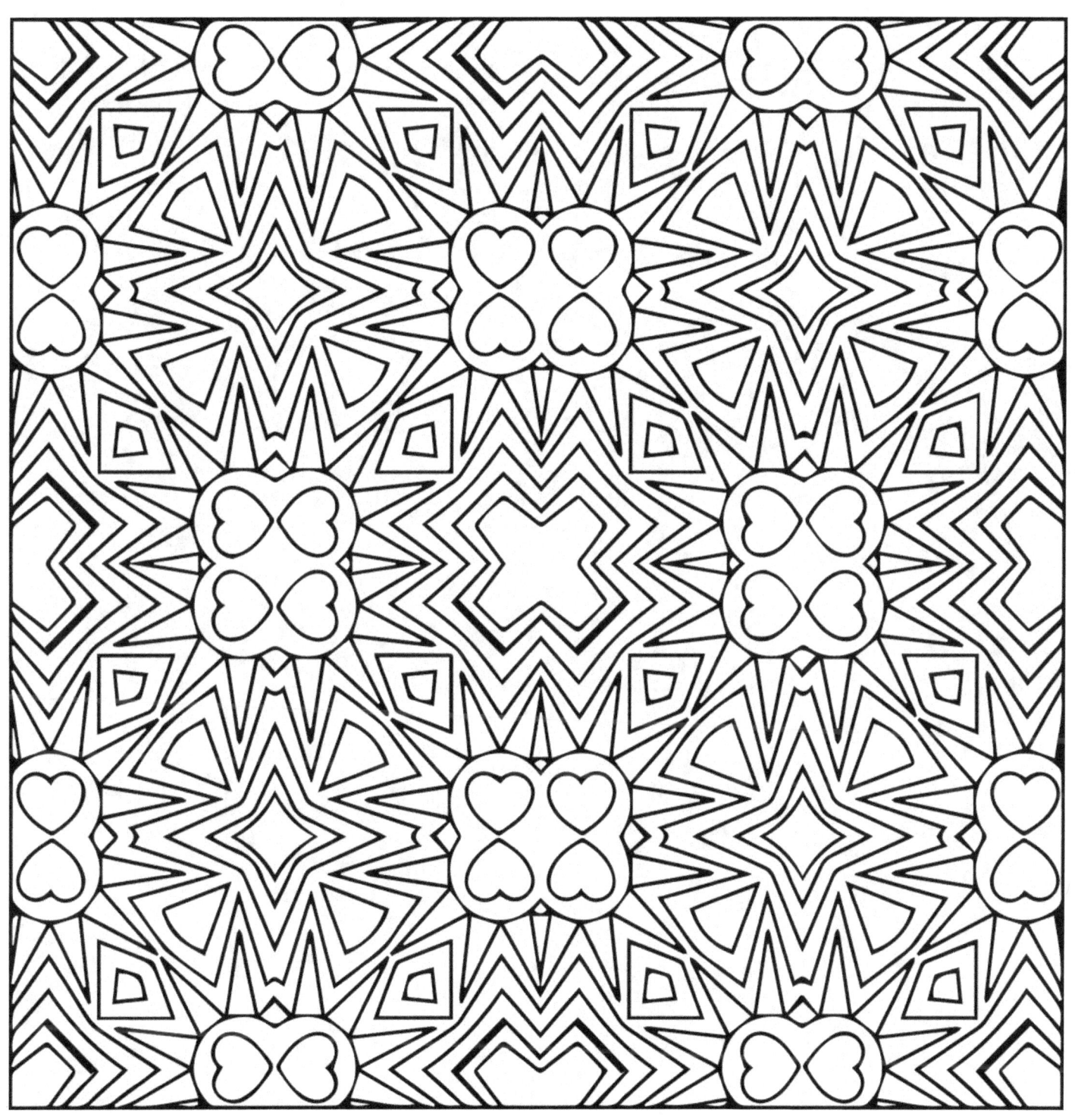

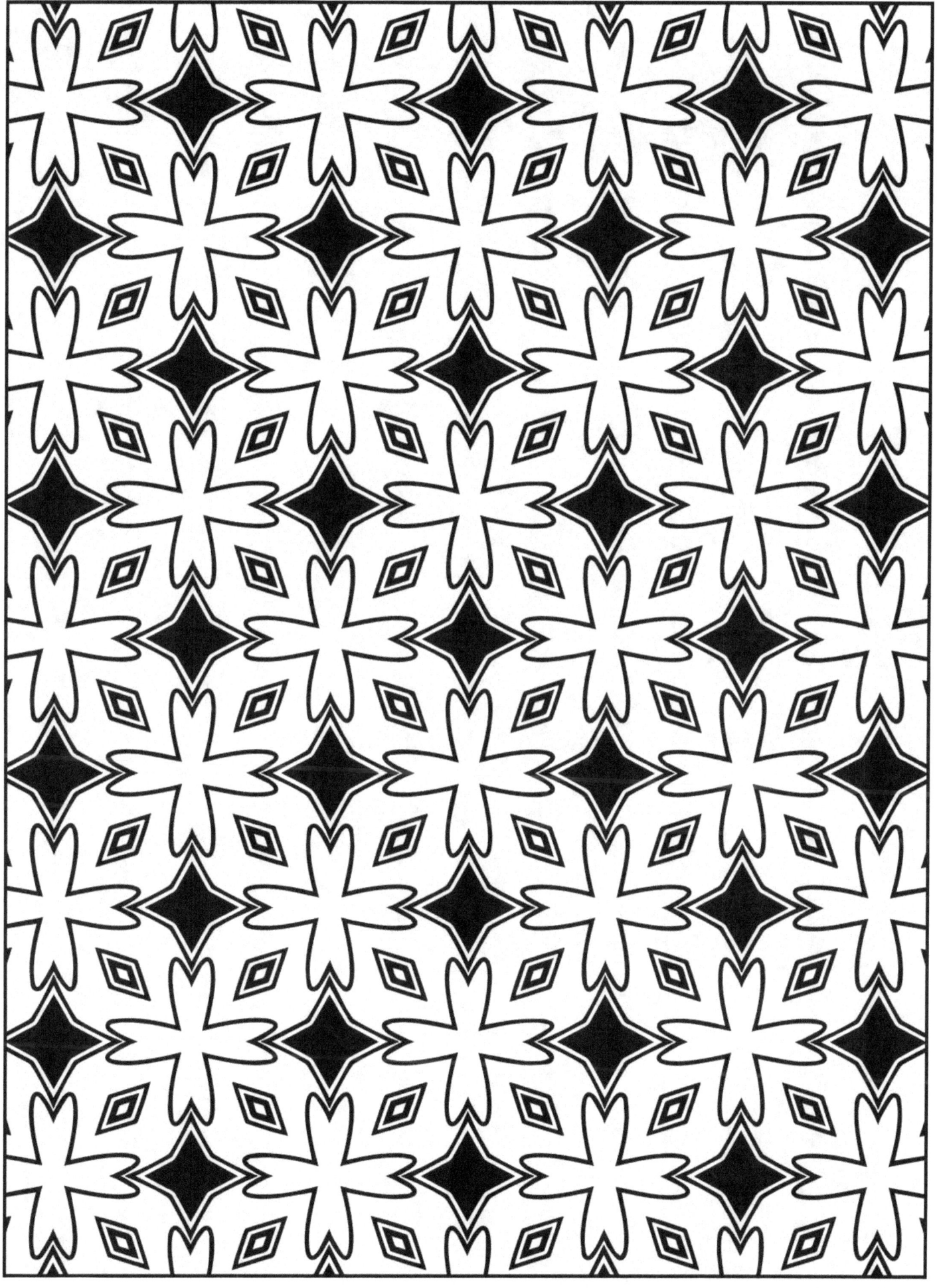

Stay In Touch & Explore More!

I hope you have enjoyed coloring this book and ask if you would please take just a moment to leave an honest review of my coloring book either on Etsy or Amazon.

I would also like to invite you to check out all of my Adult Coloring Books that are available as a paperback from Amazon here: https://amzn.to/2OK28P6 or as a PDF Digital download from my Etsy store here: https://www.etsy.com/au/shop/ColorYourWayToHappy

I love being creative and with over 40 books published so far, I'm always adding new books each month so be sure to check back and see if there's something you like.

Alternatively, if you would like to be kept up-to-date with new book releases and news please take the time to visit my Facebook page and feel free to let your friends and family know about my page too.

Don't forget to like and comment on my page and you're welcome to share your colored pages from my books there too!

Just go to: www.facebook.com/ColorYourWayToHappy

Thanks again and remember to have fun and go 'Color Your Way To Happy'!

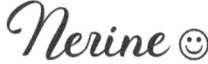

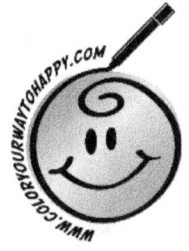